Flax Fantastic

Discover The Secret World Of Flax and exactly HOW it
will transform your health

Ken Jones

To Karen, Sarah & Nathan

Flax

"Wherever flax seed becomes a regular food item among the people, there will be better health"

– Mahatma Gandhi

Table of Contents

Introduction – Why Should You Eat Flax?

Flax seeds offer many health advantages and they are easily suitable for everyday use. The health benefits of adding flax seed to your diet are many and varied, yet it remains largely unused by the majority of the populace.

Nutritionists believe it should be an essential part of our diet. Nutritionists and food enthusiasts alike are starting to realize the important role of flax, which is also sometimes known as Linseed.

In recent decades, Americans have begun to eat far too much 'bad' fat and not nearly enough 'good' fat. This has led people to believe that eating any fat at all must be bad for them. dictum

Unfortunately, our bodies require certain amounts of balanced fats in our diets in order to maintain optimal health. Foods containing omega-3 fatty acids can actually help to balance an imbalanced diet. This is especially true of those people who tend to consume far too many omega-6 fatty acids.

While our bodies require both omega-3 and omega-6 fatty acids as essential factors of good health, recent studies by the National Institute of Health have shown that Americans tend to consume more than 10 times the amount of omega-6 fatty acids than omega-3 fatty acids. This is largely due to the high amount of processed foods in today's 'normal' diet.

This kind of imbalance can create a huge number of serious health problems, chronic diseases and health risks. The sad news is that many of these can be easily corrected and properly balanced.

Flax can play an active role in helping us to ward off health problems like heart conditions, inflammation and strokes. It even helps in the fight against cancer and diabetes, plus a number of other health benefits.

Flax can be the ideal additive into your diet to promote weight loss, as the high levels of dietary fiber can help you to feel fuller and stave of hunger pangs and food cravings.

Chapter 1 – What Is Flax?

The first question to ask is: - "What is Flax?" Flax is the seed of a blue flowering plant native to the region extending from the eastern Mediterranean to India.

Flax has been grown for thousands of years. The first known growers were in the middle-east in around 7000 BC. The main use of flax in those days was for creating linen cloth and flax oil. Over time the ancient Egyptians, Hebrews, Greeks and Romans developed the usage of flax. Flax was also cultivated throughout ancient Ethiopia. Some of these ancient cultures also used it for food and medicines. There was also a growing market for flax linen cloth for clothing and sails for ships.

By 3000 BC the Babylonians are recorded as eating flax and using oil for it's healing properties. The Romans further developed flax into bread. They also used the oil as a basis for varnish, paint and soaps.

Hippocrates is recorded and recommending flax for "mucous membrane inflammations. In the 8th century in France, Charlemagne passed laws requiring the seeds to be consumed in order to keep his subjects healthy.

The Mountain flax received its nickname of "purging flax" because it was once popular as a purgative.

Flax is full of omega-3 fatty acids, which are essential for the heart and currently a must in health advice circles. Flax seeds also contain very high levels of dietary fiber, including lignans, which are powerful anti-oxidants. It is also known to help lower cholesterol levels, which is a huge bonus in today's eating schedules.

Although flax comes in the form of seed, it can be brown or golden but the benefits to the body are exactly the same. It is surprisingly versatile. It can be used as a seed, it can be ground into flour, and it can be used in an oil form.

As a seed it will keep until needed as it is sealed inside its own shell and can be stored in an airtight container for up to a year without going rancid. The seeds can be ground in a coffee grinder or a food processor and kept ready for use in a sealed clear container in the refrigerator for up to 90 days or even frozen in a freezer. It can be used straight from the freezer as it stays in free-flowing form even when frozen. If you choose to roast the flax seed then it should also be kept in the refrigerator or freezer until needed.

Flax seed oil is slightly different to the seed form as it doesn't contain the fiber element and neither does it contain all the proteins or lignans as it does in seed form. The oil form is made by cold pressing the seed and contains mostly the fat portion of the seed. It is also important to keep it in the refrigerator and to observe the use by date, as it can have a tendency to go rancid.

Chapter 2 – What Are The Health Benefits Of Flax?

Don't let their tiny size fool you. These little seeds are packed full of vitamins, minerals, antioxidants and omega-3 fatty acids that can be enormously good for you.

There are many different health benefits to Flax seed depending on which form you use it in. As a whole seed it is very useful for its fiber content and can be sprinkled on to porridge oats or used in biscuits for its texture. However, even more benefit can come from grinding it. This is because the hard shell can be difficult to break down and so the inner nutrients can be more difficult to absorb.

Flax is suitable for all ages, although it is recommended that only a quarter of a tablespoon be given to children and toddlers as their daily intake amount. As adults we can have a lot more but it should be introduced slowly into your daily diet starting with no more than a tablespoon at most of ground or milled flax.

The health benefits flax seed oil are better than fish oil since the omega-3 found in flaxseed oil has a higher concentration of ALA. This explains what ALA means......

Our bodies can also convert ALA to EPA. But before that, the body manages to extract the goodness and health benefits of ALA that is present in flax seed oil but not fish oil. Once the ALA is converted to EPA, the body then reaps the benefits of EPA as well. This means that flaxseed oil provides better health benefits than fish oils.

However, larger amounts of flaxseed or flax seed oil should be consumed in comparison to fish oil to get the same health benefits. This is because the conversion of ALA to EPA in our bodies depends on an enzyme known as "delta-6-destaurase." This enzyme is available in varying degrees in different people. Therefore, the conversion of ALA to EPA is dependent on the adequate quantities of this enzyme that is present in our bodies. Also, the efficiency of this enzyme decreases significantly in those people who:

1. Have diabetes

2. Consume alcohol

3. Eat large quantities of fat

So, if you dislike the taste of fish oil or you do not wish to consume it, then flaxseed oil is an excellent alternative.

Health Benefits of Flax: Journal of Nutrition

A study was published in "The Journal of Nutrition" in which it was established that those who consume flaxseed oil regularly had 60% higher EPA in comparison to those who did not. An experiment was conducted for a period of 3 months on an African-American group of people who had chronic illnesses.

Every day, these people consumed flaxseed oil in the form of a capsule which provided 3 grams of ALA. The same amount of ALA can be provided by drinking 3 tablespoons of flaxseed oil. A significant number of people were tested to prove that ALA and EPA levels had risen in their bodies.

Reduction in Risk of Prostate Cancer

A researcher at Duke University, Wendy Demark-Wahnefried, was the lead author of a study which conclusively proved that a singular benefit of flax seed was the protection it afforded against the growth of cancer in the prostrate.

Research has shown that flax seeds incorporated into the diet can benefit patients with some types of breast cancer and prostate cancer by inhibiting the growth of tumors. While the study suggests that the flaxseed is able to stunt the growth of prostate tumors, further research is still being conducted.

In people who have not been diagnosed with prostate cancer, the introduction of flax into the diet can greatly reduce the risk of developing prostate cancer. The high fiber content in flax can also greatly aid digestive health and reduce inflammation, which can aggravate symptoms in people with prostate cancer.

Reduction in Severity of Symptoms in Diabetes Patients

Flaxseed also has other benefits such as diabetes prevention and treatment. Flax is able to lessen the severity of diabetes symptoms in patients with Type 2 Diabetes as it is able to assist with stabilizing blood-sugar levels. Further research is being conducted into the effects of flax on patients with Type 1 diabetes, although it is still thought to be beneficial.

The reason that flax seeds benefits us so much is because Omega 3 fatty acids are required in order to keep the walls of cells, the membranes, flexible. The function of these membranes is a lot like that of gatekeepers. They allow essential nutrients to come inside a cell and they help eliminate wastes from the cell.

Why should these cell membranes be flexible? That is because if they are flexible then, in people with diabetes, they allow better absorption of glucose in comparison to those cell membranes that are stiffer and less flexible.

Also, if the cell membranes are flexible, then they respond more efficiently to insulin. Flexible cell membranes are able to absorb glucose and insulin better even when a diabetic patient's diet is rich in saturated and hydrogenated fats.

Improved Insulin Control in Diabetes Patients

The high levels of dietary fiber found in flax seeds, coupled with so many other beneficial omega-3 fatty acids and minerals, means that people with diabetes can experience a reduction in blood sugar levels.

Research has shown that the fiber in flax can actively help to trap glucose and fat in the gut. It's able to moderate and ease the glucose release throughout the body, which effectively reduces sugar spikes. These effects have a positive impact on both blood sugar and cholesterol levels.

Reduced Risk of Colon Cancer

Studies have shown that when we consume the requisite quantities of flax seeds, then we get additional benefits as well.

For example, if Omega 3 fats are available in ample amounts in the colon, then they actually help protect the colon against cancerous cells.

If cancer causing toxins are floating around in the blood stream then Omega 3 fatty acids form a barrier and prevent these from entering the colon to a large extent. Such Omega 3 fats are also responsible for preventing dangerous and free radicals from entering our colon. This helps reduce our risks of colon cancer.

Effective Treatment of Constipation

The very high levels of dietary fiber found in flax seeds can be helpful in treating constipation. There is also support for using flax seed as a laxative, due to its fiber content. However, it's very important to drink plenty of water when adding flax into your diet, or it could result in blockages.

Fiber has long been known to help with digestion. It also helps the body to be full and to know it has had enough to eat. The presence of fiber in our diet means that our food is more satisfying and means we feel full for longer as it takes longer to digest. Fiber also helps our bodies to get rid of unwanted toxins and means we don't store so much unwanted fat in our bodies.

Reduction in Risk of Breast Cancer

Flax seeds also contain high levels of phytochemicals and phytoestrogens, including lignans, which are powerful antioxidants that could be helpful in combating free radicals within the body. It's also thought that the phytoestrogens can promote fertility and balance female hormones.

Phytoestrogens and antioxidants such as lignans have been related to effective reductions in the risk of estrogen-stimulated breast cancer. It's thought that lignan metabolites are able to bind to estrogen receptors, which can actually inhibit the onset of this type of breast cancer.

Lignans are also able to help stop the spread and growth of breast cancer even after diagnosis.

A recent study published by Clinical Cancer Research showed that women who were recently diagnosed with breast cancer were asked to consume 1 muffin per day containing 25 grams (2 tablespoons) of flaxseed. These patients showed a significant reduction in tumor growth as compared to those patients who ate muffins containing no flax at all.

Further studies have shown that the addition of flax into the diet slowed the rate of tumor growth. The research proved that eating flax regularly in the daily diet can help reduce the risk of metastasis and improve the clinical prognosis of breast cancer. It's also proven to reduce and even stop the risk of a patient contracting hormone-related breast cancer after menopause by up to 30%.

Reduction in Risk of Heart Disease

Omega 3 fats that are found in flax and flax seeds are one of the key ingredients that are used by our bodies to produce those elements that help eliminate blood clots. Clots in our blood stream lead to heart diseases andstrokes. This actually helps reduce the risks that we have for getting a debilitating heart attack or even atherosclerosis.

Improvement in Heart Health

Studies reported by the MayoClinic.com show that people who have suffered heart attacks show very positive health results after adding flax seeds into their diets. Flax seed can reduce the level of LDL (bad cholesterol) in the system as well as reducing total blood cholesterol levels.

Lignans also work to help increase the HDL (good cholesterol) levels within the cardiovascular system, which is beneficial in reducing the risk of heart disease. As LDL levels are reduced, the fat that can build up in arteries is reduced, which in turn reduces the risk of heart attack or stroke.

However, flax seed also contains properties that can reduce inflammation. Patients with atherosclerosis, or 'hardening of the arteries', are usually affected by high cholesterol levels coupled with inflammation.

Recent studies show that patients with atherosclerosis can benefit from taking flax seed for its ability to help reduce cholesterol and reduce inflammation simultaneously.

The high natural levels of lignans, dietary fiber, and omega-3 fatty acids mean that this combination could play a major part in helping to prevent heart disease.

According to the National Institutes of Health (NIH), the majority of American diets no longer contain the amount of omega-3 fatty acids required in our daily diets to sustain health and wellness.

It's been found that many Americans now consume more than 10 times the amount of omega-6 fatty acids than omega-3 fatty acids. While Omega-6 fatty acid is another essential fat required by the body, taken in excess it can contribute to heart problems and obesity problems.

Therefore the research concludes that adding flax seeds, containing health omega-3 fatty acids, can help to correct these imbalances. Once stabilized, there is a significant reduction in the risk of many chronic diseases noticed in almost all patients.

Reduction in Inflammation

Inflammation is now recognized medically as a type of nonspecific immune response that is thought to be the underlying factor in many chronic diseases and illnesses.

The high levels of Omega-3 fatty acids found in flaxseeds are thought to be a key element in fighting inflammation within the body. Research shows that inflammation plays an integral part in chronic diseases like heart disease, arthritis, asthma, diabetes and even some forms of cancer.

In fact, inflammation may be behind much of what ails us. Research has shown that uncontrolled inflammation can be an underlying factor in most health problems. The white blood cells, which release large amounts of inflammation-causing substances, do play a role in damaging arterial walls, which can set the stage for cholesterol deposits and heart disease.

Your body makes C-reactive Protein from interleukin-6, which is a very strong inflammation-causing immune chemical. This chemical is a cell communication molecule and it tells your immune system wrongfully that it needs to go into full defense mode, releasing C-reactive Protein that then causes inflammation.

Research published by the New England Journal of Medicine showed that people with very high C-reactive Protein levels were 4 and a half times more likely to suffer a heart attack. This makes C-reactive Protein readings far more accurate than cholesterol readings for specialists predicting heart attack risks.

Unfortunately, high C-reactive Protein levels are also found in people with type 2 diabetes and in overweight patients with pre-diabetes symptoms. Once again, the C-reactive Protein levels are indicators of inflammation levels.

Being overweight or obese can also increase inflammation. This is because the adipose cells, particularly those around the tummy, will produce large amounts of interleukin-6 and C-reactive Protein, which cause more inflammation.

Infection can also be made much worse in patients already struggling to control inflammation. When tissue becomes infected by bacteria, the white blood cells migrate to the site of the infection and begin to ingest the bacteria. Unfortunately, the bacteria will thrive and multiply within the white cells. The white cells then burst, releasing more bacteria into the tissue and releasing C-reactive Protein into the surrounding tissue. This results in even more inflammation, especially as more white cells will swarm to the area in an effort to try and combat the infection.

Long term, or chronic, inflammation also has a detrimental effect on bone density, which can weaken them and even shrink them. Inflammation-related bone loss is a major clinical problem that can occur in various diseases, including periodontal disease, osteoarthritis, rheumatoid arthritis and some types of osteoporosis.

Studies show that inflammation in patients with the chronic diseases and ailments noted above could be enhanced by insufficient Omega-3 fatty acid intake. Yet patients who introduced flax seeds into their diet show an improvement in the levels of inflammation. People without these diseases can effectively reduce their risk of contracting them by eating flax.

This is really big news in the health world as we are all supposed to eat more of this fatty acid. It helps to fight disease and corrects imbalances in the body due to eating "bad" fats that are harder for our bodies to absorb. It is even thought that the Omega 3 in flaxseed is more beneficial than the Omega 3 found in fish – a definite benefit for Vegans and those who do not eat fish!

Omega 3 fatty acids are known to be a cholesterol buster and having Flaxseed in your regular intake of food can help to lower your cholesterol levels – a must for those with high blood pressure and diabetes.

One of the types of antioxidants present in Flaxseed in very high levels is lignans. These are natural antioxidants that help to slow the activity of cell damaging free radicals in our bodies. Basically, they appear to improve our general well being and slow the aging process. In effect , we are taking in a natural product that can help in the battle against cancer, menopause, artery problems, and both type 1 & type 2 Diabetes.

Reduction in Depression

Research has shown that depression could be inextricably linked to an overactive immune system and inflammation.

Most people associate depression with being run down and having poor immunity. However, the surprising side-effects noticed by researchers using immune-boosting drugs show that some people could actually be experiencing depression due to an over-active immune system.

The studies showed that by reducing the level of inflammation within patients, the symptoms of depression are significantly reduced. In some patients it was noticed that the depression had subsided completely.

Researchers now believe that working to reduce inflammation could offer a brand new way to treat routine clinical depression effectively without the need for pharmaceutical drugs.

The key to this research lies in understanding how the immune system reacts in the presence of infection, thus stimulating inflammation and causing dark moods to arise in patients.

Studies conducted by a psychiatrist in the University of Maastricht in the Netherlands first showed the connection between mood and inflammation back in 1990. Since that time it's been widely recognized that people suffering from depression are often also unusually vulnerable to infections and cancer.

While some researchers initially believed this link was a result of an under-performing immune system, it's since been found that the immune cells were more active than normal, not under-active.

People with depression often show raised body temperatures, which does suggest that they suffer from a form of chronic inflammation. People diagnosed with clinical depression are also three times more likely to die of heart disease, which is usually caused by arteriosclerosis (an inflammation of the lining of the arteries).

Yet even though these findings have been recognized for a couple of decades, they have gone largely ignored by the multi-billion dollar pharmaceutical industry until recently.

Researchers have shown that patients who add 2 tablespoons of flaxseed into their diets daily show a significant improvement in depression symptoms. This is because of the anti-inflammatory properties within flax, treating the underlying inflammation problems and thus correcting the imbalance that creates the depression.

Reducing Cholesterol Levels

In another study, 40 patients with high cholesterol were examined. Each of these people had cholesterol levels that were in excess of 240 mg/dL. One group continued with their regular statin drugs and the other group was given 20g of flax seeds every day for sixty day. At the end of the trial period, both groups were examined for factors such as cholesterol, triglycerides, LDL cholesterol, HDL cholesterol and so on.

The good news was that the group that consumed flax seeds showed the same amount of improvement as the group that had continued with their statin drugs!

This proves that flax seed benefit us as much as statin drugs do! The table below gives the exact benefits of flax seeds that were demonstrated in that study:

	Measured Factors	Significant Reductions
1	Total Cholesterol	-17.20%
2	LDL Cholesterol	-3.90%
3	Triglycerides	-36.30%
4	Ratio of Total Cholesterol / HDL Cholesterol	-33.50%

Table 1: Flax Seeds Benefits: Lower Cholesterol

These readings were determined after examining the group at the beginning of the study period and at the end of the sixty day trial period. The group that had continued with their statin drugs displayed almost the same readings and the benefits did not differ significantly between both groups.

Controls Blood Pressure in Patients with High Cholesterol

In a study conducted over three months, a group of researchers in Greek examined the systolic and diastolic blood pressure of about sixty middle aged men. One group of these people consumed safflower oil and the other groups consumed flaxseed oil regularly, as part of their daily diet.

The flaxseed oil that the group consumed in their diet provided them with ALA (Alpha Linolenic Acid) of 8 grams. Our bodies process flaxseed oil in to ALA, DHA and EPA (EicosaPentaenoic Acid). The group that consumed safflower oil, had effectively eaten LA (Linolenic Acid) of 11 grams on a daily basis. Safflower oil is known to be a concentrated source of Omega 6 fats.

At the end of sixty days, it was seen that the group that consumed the Omega 3 rich flaxseed oil had significantly lower systolic and diastolic blood pressure in comparison to the other group.

This was considered to be startling news since both, Omega 3 and Omega 6 are essential fats: we need both these fatty acids to survive and to be healthy! We must eat both these types of fats in our diets. Then the question remains that why did the group that consumed flaxseed oil only display lowered blood pressure?

Reduction in High Blood Pressure

Studies have also shown that people with high blood pressure also benefit from flax seeds. In a research conducted for INTERMAP, the International Study of Macro- and Micro-nutrients and Blood Pressure, data was analyzed in which it was revealed that people who consume more flax seeds benefit substantially because their blood pressure is lower than those who don't consume flax.

This team of researchers found that people who absorbed Omega 3 fats from certain foods had lowered their blood pressure as much as those who ate fish in order to introduce Omega 3 fats in their system.

Apart from fish, the foods that lowered their blood pressure included the following:

Nuts

Seeds

Vegetable oils, for example, walnuts

Flaxseed

This study was headed by H Ueshima and others, and Ueshima has stated, ""With blood pressure, every millimeter counts. The effect of each nutrient is apparently small but independent, so together they can add up to a substantial impact on blood pressure. If you can reduce blood pressure by a few ms by:

Eating less salt

Losing a few pounds

Avoiding heavy drinking

Eating more:

Vegetables

Whole grains and

Fruits

(for their fiber, minerals, vegetable protein and other nutrients)

and getting more Omega 3 fatty acids, then you've made a big difference."

Reduction in ADHD Symptoms

Research conducted at the MayoClinic.com shows that people with ADHD (Attention Deficit Hyperactivity Disorder) may have deficiencies or imbalances in certain unsaturated fatty acids like omega-3 fatty acids. These deficiencies or imbalances may be a contributing factor in ADHD and the associated symptoms.

Most people diagnosed with ADHD show signs of inattention, hyperactivity and impulsivity as key behaviors. Some of the predominant inattentive type symptoms may include being easily distracted, being forgetful and becoming very bored with a task after a short time. The hyperactive symptoms tend to include fidgeting, impatience, interrupting others, incessant talking and having difficulty in doing quiet tasks.

Research has shown that many people diagnosed with ADHD may have accompanying disorders, such as anxiety or depression. These combinations make it very difficult to treat patients effectively using pharmaceutical medications.

However, the studies also suggest that adding omega-3 fatty acids in the form of flax seeds can improve the symptoms of ADHD significantly. Since the link to the immune system, inflammation and depression was ascertained, researchers determined that some forms of ADHD may also hold similar links and be based on an over-active immune system, leading to inflammation and behavioral issues.

Improvement in Psoriasis Symptoms

Psoriasis is a chronic autoimmune disease that affects the skin. The immune system begins to send out incorrect signals to the body to speed up the growth of skin cells. This is often displayed as red, scaly patches on the skin and they are known to be an inflammation of excessive skin production.

Many patients with psoriasis become self-conscious and suffer reduced confidence levels as they fear how others will perceive their scaly skin condition. Yet psoriasis is not contagious.

Treatments for psoriasis include various topical treatments, such as bath solutions, moisturizers, mineral oils and petroleum jelly. There are also wide ranges of medicated creams and ointments available to try and alleviate some of the symptoms. Unfortunately, many of these medicated creams may irritate normal skin, even while they're helping to address the psoriasis affected skin areas.

Phototherapy, or ultraviolet light treatment, has also been used with some limited success in psoriasis patients. Exposure to sunlight can help to reduce and improve psoriasis in some patients.

Studies on patients show a significant improvement in the severity of psoriasis after introducing flax into their diets. As psoriasis is an inflammatory condition, the lignans found within flax go to work with their anti-inflammatory properties and help to reduce the outbreaks of psoriasis.

Reduction in Eczema Symptoms

While eczema is not a life-threatening disease, it can be awfully annoying to people who have it. Some people have embarrassing red, scaly skin on their hands, feet or faces, while other people may find their eczema is easier to disguise beneath clothing on other parts of their body.

Eczema is form of dermatitis, which is caused by inflammation of the epidermis (the outer layer of the skin).

Specialists are unable to cure eczema with medical treatment, yet they continue to prescribe corticosteroids as treatment for eczema patients. These corticosteroids are often powerful anti-inflammatory drugs designed to reduce the level of inflammation on the skin.

Prolonged use of topical corticosteroids can have side effects. These include the skin becoming thin and fragile. Additionally, if topical corticosteroid treatments are used over large areas, there is a risk that an amount may be absorbed into the body, which can cause hypothalamic-pituitary-adrenal axis suppression, resulting in negative affects to the immune system, digestion, mood and emotion and sexuality.

However, patients consuming small quantities of flax seed in their diet have noticed a significant improvement in the amount of eczema they display on their skin. The red, inflamed patches begin to reduce quite rapidly and the itching is almost completely stopped. New outbreaks of eczema are much less frequent.

As flax seeds contain such powerful anti-inflammatory properties, this could become a natural way to treat eczema and dermatitis without the need to use potentially harmful corticosteroidal treatments.

Reduction in Symptoms for IBD and Crohn's Disease

Recent studies have concluded that there is a positive connection between patients taking flax seed and the reduction in the severity of symptoms for IBD (inflammatory bowel disease or ulcerative colitis) and Crohn's disease. The study shows that the inner lining of the intestines is inflamed during the worst symptoms, yet after adding flax seed into the diet, patients show very little to no inflammation within the inner lining of the intestines, leading to a major reduction in symptoms.

Inflammatory bowel disease is an inflammatory disease of the large intestine, or colon. The inner lining of the intestine becomes inflamed and develops ulcers. This is often the most severe in the rectal area, which can cause frequent bouts of diarrhea. Mucus and blood often appear in the feces if the lining becomes damaged.

Crohn's disease is different to IBD in that it affects a different part of the bowel. Usually people with Crohn's disease are affected by inflammation within the lining of the small intestine (terminal ileum) and only parts of the large intestine. Crohn's disease often causes a much deeper level of inflammation that extends into the layers of the intestinal wall.

Flax has a strong tendency to reduce inflammation and aid digestive health overall. Patients with IBD and Crohn's disease report greatly reduced symptoms after adding 2 tablespoons of flax into their diet daily. Add this important anti-inflammatory function to the natural levels of high dietary fiber and it's easy to see why people who suffer with IBD and Crohn's disease can benefit from flax.

Reduction in Inflammation-Related Asthma Symptoms

Asthma is strongly linked to inflammation of the bronchial tubes that constrict and narrow the breathing passageways. Asthma sufferers know all too well the difficulty in breathing in enough air or letting it back out again without that familiar wheeze and often an accompanying pain in the chest, for some patients.

Untreated asthma can be fatal and many asthma specialists will prescribe very strong anti-inflammatory medication in an attempt to reduce the inflammation within the bronchial tubes and bring the asthma back under control.

Many asthma patients are prescribed with inhalers that act as relievers and preventers in an attempt to keep the inflammation under control. These inhalers usually consist of a Salbutamol inhaler (i.e. Ventolin or Airomir or Aerolin) and a corticosteroid inhaler containing budesonide (i.e. Sybmicort or Pulmicort).

While these inhalers work effectively to control the symptoms of asthma in most patients, they are known for some common side effects.

Potential side effects for salbutamol include tremors, headaches, muscle cramps and heart palpitations. Some of the more severe symptoms can include tachycardia (rapid heart rate), hypotension and collapse, especially after large doses.

Potential side effects for the strong corticosteroids like budesonide include headache, sore throat, dizziness, stomach pain, stuffy nose, tremors and vomiting. Some of the more severe symptoms can include seizures, chest pain and fast or irregular heartbeat.

While asthma patients will still require their medications, any attempt to reduce dependence on this medication will be seen as positive by an asthma specialist.

Trials using flax seeds in the diet of asthma patients have shown a marked improvement in asthma symptoms. Many of those patients reported a reduced need to be reliant on medication, while others reported far fewer incidences of wheezing and shortness of breath.

This is thought to be based on the anti-inflammatory properties of flax seed helping to keep the level of inflammation in the bronchial tubes more under control.

Improved Fertility and Reduced Menopausal Symptoms

Research has shown that patients who have introduced flax seeds into their diets can experience a reduction in peri-menopausal symptoms. Reports indicate that women who include flax in their diet experience an improvement in the level of premenstrual breast pain and tenderness as well as a reduction in the severity of menstrual cramps.

The lignans found in flax seeds are also thought to promote fertility and are known to help deter pre-term labor. These same phytoestrogens are also able to block tumor formation, which offers protection against hormone-sensitive cancers, such as breast cancer, ovarian cancer, endometrium and prostate cancer.

In women of menopausal age, the reduced estrogen levels within their bodies can create well-known symptoms such as hot flashes, migraine, rapid heartbeat, back pain, depression, dry skin, fatigue, frequent urination, sleep disturbance, itching, cramps and moodiness.

However, one of the most notable symptoms is the increased susceptibility menopausal women have to inflammation and infection.

Many women are prescribed with pharmaceutical drugs for hormone replacement therapy in an effort to counteract these symptoms. Yet patients who have added flaxseed into their diets report greatly reduced symptoms and far less complications due to inflammation.

The high level of the powerful anti-oxidants called lignans found within flax seed actively help to act as a phyto-estrogen. This can help to correct the imbalance in falling estrogen levels naturally and counteract the effect of menopause.

Chapter 3 - Omega-3 Fatty Acid and ALA

Flaxseeds have a distinct nutty flavor of their own and they also have omega-3 fatty acids which make these seeds very popular with those who are health conscious. In fact, the omega-3 fatty acids that are prevalent in flaxseeds are critical for good health.

It contains Alpha Linolenic Acid (ALA) which is also the precursor of the omega-3 fatty acid that is found in food such as fish oils. The specific omega-3 found in fish oils is known as Eicosapentaenoic Acid (EPA).

The Importance of Omega-3 Fatty Acids Present within Flax

Why is Omega-3 so important to our well-being? Omega-3 fatty acids have several anti-inflammatory properties which are required in order to reduce the inflammation associated with various diseases such as:

Asthma

Osteoarthritis

Osteoporosis

Rheumatoid arthritis

Migraines and headaches

When we consume Omega-3 fatty acids, then our bodies produce prostaglandins, that are substances which are quite similar to hormones and these are made from fatty acids. Series 1 and Series 3 prostaglandins contain molecules that are anti-inflammatory in nature. In contrast, Series 2 prostaglandins have molecules that are pro-inflammatory in nature and these are available in Omega-6 fats.

Omega-6 fats are found in:

Margarine

Animal fats

Soy

Vegetable oils like corn, palm, safflower, peanut and sunflower oils The Fine Balance of Omega 3 and Omega 6 Fatty Acids

The answer is simple: Omega 3 fats have anti-inflammatory properties. This helps control blood pressure. However, when we consume lesser quantities of Omega 3 fats, then the Omega 6 fats promote inflammation in our bodies. All Omega 6 fats need to be balanced by the requisite quantities of Omega 3 fats.

What is the correct proportion of Omega 3 and Omega 6 fats in our bodies? Unfortunately, at this point in time there is no consensus on this matter. Many experts will tell you that Omega 6: Omega 3 ratio should be no more than 4:1. Other experts firmly believe that this ratio should be 2:1. But, across the board, all nutrition experts know for a fact that when there is an imbalance of these fats in our bodies then Omega 6 fats cannot, by themselves, fight off diseases such as blood pressure and cholesterol.

In order to get the maximum protection against heart diseases, it is important to retain this delicate balance. The bad news is that most diets in the Western world are not able to keep this balance. A typical American diet, for example, provides a shocking amount of 10 times more Omega 6 fats that Omega 3 fats! Therefore, in order to improve your odds, you must increase the amounts of Omega 3 in your diet.

You can retain the balance of Omega 3 and Omega 6 fats in your diet by eating foods that are rich in Omega 3 like:

Flaxseed oil

Canola oil

Walnuts

Cold water fish, for example, wild salmon and so on.

On the other hand, Omega 6 fats are derived from sources such as:

Safflower oil

Corn oil

Peanut oil

Butter and

Meats

This doesn't mean you stop eating butter or meat altogether. This study merely says that you should be able to retain the requisite proportions of Omega 6: Omega 3 fats in your system so that you can ward off diseases such as blood pressure or high cholesterol more effectively.

Healthy Bones and Reduction of Bone Loss

Omega 3 fat that is found in flax also provides other benefits. For example, it promotes the health of your bones and reduces bone loss. The specific Omega 3 fat is known as "Alpha linolenic acid" and this is found in flax seeds as well as in walnuts. When there is an imbalance in our bodies of the proportions of Omega 3 and Omega 6 fat, then Alpha linolenic acid helps avert extreme amounts of bone turnover, according to the "Nutrition Journal."

Other studies have also been conducted in which researchers have established the fact that if we include rich amounts of Omega 3 in our diets, for example by eating fish, then this helps reduce bone loss. Scientists believe that this is because our bodies convert Omega 3 acids into anti-inflammatory prostaglandins and Omega 6 fats into pro-inflammatory prostaglandins.

Therefore, you can protect your bones, make them stronger and prevent bone loss by including the following in your diet:

Nuts

Cold Water Fish

Walnuts

Flaxseeds (since they are rich in anti-inflammatory Omega-3 fatty acids)

Also, researchers have noticed that if people consume a diet that is rich in Omega 3 fats, then their bodies have much higher levels of "TNF alpha" or Tumour Necrosis Factor-alpha. This is a marker of inflammation and it correlates to the level of N-telopeptides in our bodies.

The health benefits of flax are not only confined to bone density and anti-inflammation. Health benefits of flax also include protection against inflammatory-related diseases such as diabetes, cancer as well as heart problems.

Powerhouse of Vitamins and Minerals

Flaxseed also contains a wide array of vitamins and minerals in natural form. This includes Vitamin E, VitaminB-6, copper, Zinc, Magnesium, Potassium, and folate. All together these combine with the other ingredients found in flaxseed to make it a very beneficial part of our daily diet. Together they aid our bodies in their fight to maintain our health. They improve our stamina, which is a must for athletes as well as our everyday living demands, help our bodies to get good benefits from our foods and weed out the bad. It means people with both Type 1 and Type 2 diabetes have a natural ally in the fight to maintain healthy insulin levels.

In this modern age when people are wary of taking more and more medication to ward off heart issues like blood pressure, dietary concerns like being overweight , even help in recovering from surgery or cancer treatments, it is good to learn about natural ingredients that our bodies can absorb easily to improve and maintain our health and general well-being.

Flax Secret 1

Why Eating too Much Flax is Dangerous: How Much is Enough?

There are no recorded flax seed oil side effects that inflicted harm on humans. Nevertheless, moderation is necessary. Flaxseed may have side effects when consumed in large quantities, especially if it is uncooked. Flaxseed contains cynogenic glycosides and in uncooked flaxseed intakes amounting to more than 10 tablespoons the cyanide level may reach to toxic levels.

Large amount intake of flaxseed may upset hormonal balance. Studies on animals have reported birth defects. However, there is no reported danger of flaxseed on pregnancy or children. Most studies that reported a health benefit by eating flaxseed used no more than 2 tablespoons per day for adults.

Chapter 4 - What Are the Different Forms of Flax?

There are 2 main types of flax seed. One is primarily used for making linen and cloths. The other is used for the flax oil and seeds.

The largest 2 flax producers in the world are Canada and The Republic Of China. Modern farming techniques have developed flax to the point that most climates that have a reasonable amount of rainfall. Here in the UK you can often see fields of blue flax flowers in fields alongside the bright yellow rape seed fields. It looks stunning and surreal but also very beautiful.

If you also wish to also take advantage of the health benefits of flax, then you can consume these in a variety of different ways, for example you can consider:

Whole flaxseeds: these have a soft crunchy texture

Ground flaxseeds: the nutrients in these are more easily consumed than whole flaxseeds

Flaxseed oil

Flaxseeds are distinctive in appearance; if you recollect sesame seeds, then flaxseeds are slightly larger in dimension than them. They have a shinier and smoother outer shell which is hard to touch. The color of flaxseeds ranges from a deep amber shade to a brownish red color. You will be able to buy flaxseeds that are of two varieties: brown or golden.

Both brown and golden flax are good for you. A team of scientists from the Scientific Institute for the Study of flaxseed, from Canada and the US, have conducted multiple studies on the health benefits of flax. They have established its role in the prevention as well as the curing of several degenerative diseases, along with many other health benefits related to the reduction in risk of contracting multiple diseases and disorders.

How Do These Different Forms of Flax Help You?

Aside from the noticeable health benefits derived from consuming flax, the different forms of flax can have other benefits too. These include anti-aging benefits and increases in skin tone.

It's long been established that the anti-aging industry works to try and reduce the signs of aging on a person's skin, which is the first place most people associate with trying to hold back the years. Yet researchers are very well aware that a reduction in inflammation can significantly improve skin tone.

Effects of Aging and Inflammation

Inflammation is a vital defense mechanism of your body designed for survival. Unfortunately, uncontrolled chronic inflammation can contribute to degenerative diseases, disorders and an increase in the speed of the aging process.

Ideally, inflammation is designed to clear out any infection within your body and then subside so that normal tissue can be rebuilt. During a bout of inflammation, there is an increase in localized blood flow, activation of the immune cells in the affected area, release of large quantities of free radicals, destruction of healthy or normal tissue and deposits of scar tissue. When the infection is over, the inflammation is supposed to subside.

Yet inflammation is capable of remaining even long after the initial infection is gone, sometimes for months or even years. This is known as chronic inflammation and usually occurs because the inflammation response has become sensitive or because the immune system begins to perceive some of your own body's tissue as being foreign.

Because of these issues, aging is strongly associated with the increase in chronic inflammation. As our bodies grow older, we tend to develop autoimmune conditions that can stimulate more inflammation.

While the medical world focuses on how inflammation can affect your heart, your arteries, your immune system, your digestive system and your overall health, there is one factor that has been largely left forgotten – your skin.

Chronic inflammation is known to play a significant role in skin aging. However, oxidization can also play a part in skin losing its firmness and youthful appearance. This is where wrinkles begin to form.

Many anti-wrinkle creams and lotions contain anti-oxidants, but these are placed on top of your skin. Only a very small amount of those creams actually seeps into the deeper layers of your skin where the damage is really being done.

In order to really combat the effects of aging skin and wrinkles, it's important to work from the inside out. Reducing inflammation and increasing the anti-oxidants you consume can help to rejuvenate tired, wrinkled skin by offering it more hydration and by replenishing damaged cells.

Fortunately, flax seeds contain great anti-inflammatory properties as well as very powerful anti-oxidants that could be the key to your anti-aging efforts There are a number of good things that will happen to your skin when you eat flax. Most people find a huge improvement in the condition of their skin. It becomes smoother and hydrated. The Omega-3 fatty acids also accelerate the skin's own natural healing process.

Flax contains anti-inflammatory properties, which means that if you suffer from skin rashes, psoriasis, acne and eczema you could find an improvement in these conditions.

There is, however, a problem with assuming that eating flax will change your skin condition for the better. Most people will find their conditions and skin problem improve as a natural result of eating flax. There are some chronic sufferers that find their conditions worsen with flax. You will need to check with your doctor if you are in any doubt about this aspect.

There are a number of good things that will happen to your skin when you eat flax. Most people find a huge improvement in the condition of their skin. It becomes smoother and hydrated. The Omega-3 fatty acids also accelerate the skin's own natural healing process.

Flax contains anti-inflammatory properties, which means that if you suffer from skin rashes, psoriasis, acne and eczema you could find an improvement in these conditions.

There is, however, a problem with assuming that eating flax will change your skin condition for the better. Most people will find their conditions and skin problem improve as a natural result of eating flax. There are some chronic sufferers that find their conditions worsen with flax. You will need to check with your doctor if you are in any doubt about this aspect.

As well as eating flax there are moisturizers and skin creams that contain flax. Then there is pure flax oil itself which you can apply to your skin. For the most part you will find that you will notice a great improvement to your skin. There are three main areas where you will see improvements.

Flax Provides Protection

The protection is provided by that fact that your skin condition is more hydrated and everyday irritants will not affect you nearly as severely. You will build up a resistance to plants that normally affect you with allergenic properties and this can help reduce redness or irritation that occurs on the skin upon contact with these pollens.

Flax Gives Great Skin Tone

Because flax helps prevent your skin from drying out it has a chance to heal quickly and maintain its balance. Cell reproduction will stabilize and become normal and the risk of dry skin disorders is reduced. There is a well known "glow" that your skin will have if it never has the chance to dry out.

Flax Maintains Hydration

Further to the improved skin tone is the added benefit of being well hydrated. You will find you skin smoother because of the fact that it is always well hydrated. This extra level of hydration can also help you if you happen to get sunburned. Your skin will be able to repair itself much faster if you have been eating flax.

Chapter 5 - How Flax Helps With A Weight Loss Diet

As many people have found out to their cost, dieting makes you fat. You start out with good intentions and reduce your intake of fatty foods and processed foods. You will be following the latest diet guru's book in your quest to lose weight. You have your weight targets and for the first 2 weeks all goes well.

Then something inside begins to change. Your body starts to realize that maybe you are not eating what it is used to. So it decides you need some help and goes into famine mode. You body's metabolism slows down and every possible ounce of nutrition is absorbed to preserve your life.

So your own body can turn against you and slow down your weight loss dramatically once it realizes that you are eating less. This is when your body goes into survival mode.

You see, when you diet, you're consuming far less calories than you were before the diet. Your body doesn't know what's going on. It just assumes you're starving. So rather than start shedding that excess fat, your body stores it to help protect you against a famine. This makes it awfully hard to get that weight off.

There is also a second problem with of the shelf processed foods that are low in fat or even fat free. These food products are highly processed and are packed with carbohydrates. So your body works against you again and the production of insulin increases. Your body also converts much of that carbohydrate into fat as it recognizes that your fat intake is very low.

This process will continue until you have what is known as a "Pizza Day Crash". You come to a day when you feel the only food that will satisfy you is a fat-filled pizza. For pizza you can also substitute chocolate, fried fish and chips, or any other fat encompassing junk food, but the result will be almost exactly the same.

Your body starts to scream out for some fatty acids to help it survive. The problem is that your body cannot use these foods to convert into the valuable omega-3 oils it is looking for. It simply continues to store them as more of the fat you're trying so hard to get rid of.

So the right thing to do in order to get your body into a condition where it will begin to shift that stubborn fat is to add essential fatty acids to your diet to replace the shortage that your body is feeling. Omega-3 fatty acids and omega-6 fatty acids in the right balanced amounts can actually help to increase your metabolism and make it much easier for you to begin losing weight properly.

There are many excellent and natural sources of these essential fatty acids including egg yolks, poultry, green leafy vegetables, nuts and certain types of fruit. The highest concentration of omega-3 fatty acids in plants is found in flax seeds.

Flax is unique in having this very high amount of essential fatty acids contained within the seeds. This includes all colors of flax seeds. There are some minor variables in the nutritional content between varieties but nothing significant. The point is that if you can find a way to add flax seed to your diet on a daily basis then your body will not have these feelings of famine. Consequently you will not crave more food or the wrong food and your weight loss will continue.

One further point about the essential fatty acids in flax is that it does not convert into body fat in your body. It is safe to eat and will remove the cravings you associate with dieting. One of the many problems with the modern diet is that most people never eat enough of these essential fatty acids even when they are overeating.

Yet they'll consume more than 10 times the amount that they need in 'bad' fats instead. These types of foods are usually processed foods, fast food or fatty junk food filled with calories but containing very little nutritional value. This means you can eat and eat, but still not quite feel satisfied, which usually means eating more.

So you could easily consume 4000 or 5000 calories per day and still feel hungry. How crazy is that?

Yet adding a simple thing, like 2 tablespoons of flax into your diet each day can reduce the likelihood of this happening. The high levels of dietary fiber in flax make you feel fuller and more satisfied, while the healthy addition of omega-3 fatty acids in your diet can help to correct the imbalances caused by eating too much of the wrong types of fat.

There are secondary weight loss benefits to eating flax too. The main one being that over time the hard fats you have accumulated over time will be removed and excreted. This is not a short term process but is very tangible. If you eat flax for 30 days you can sense the changes in your body make up and enjoy the benefits of being lighter and fitter.

Another bonus is that it becomes much easier to exercise as you do not feel bloated and heavy. You are much more inclined to go for a walk if you are feeling the energy burst you get from eating flax and losing weight. This is what I call a virtuous circle. Doing one good thing, eating flax, means that you automatically take other actions that are positive for your overall health. It's a classic win-win situation.

How you actually include flax into your diet is up to you. Flax comes in a number of forms but by far the most beneficial is flax meal, sometimes called ground flax. You can use a small coffee grinder to grind the seeds into a light powder. You can add this to breakfast cereals, juices and bean salads. Other people simply add it to a glass of water and drink it.

The only problem is if you don't like the nutty taste of flax you might prefer to mask the flax flavor with other foods. Of course, you also have the option of learning to make simple recipes that enhance that nutty flavor and make it into an essential part of that dish.

You must not overdo your consumption of flax and most nutritionist say that a recommended amount for adults is 2 tablespoon per day. Even at this seemingly small amount, it's very possible to see great results in your health and your overall well-being.

Flax Secret 2

How Flax Can Transform Your Health If You Don't Eat Meat Or Fish

It is even thought that the high levels in Omega-3 fatty acids found in flaxseed are more beneficial than the Omega-3 fatty acids found in fish. This can be a definite benefit for Vegans and those who do not eat fish!

The biggest challenge for vegans is trying to replace eggs in some recipes. Eggs are used to bind, they leaven and they give structure to baked goods. Yet flax seeds can become a very healthy egg-replacement that works very well.

Simply mix 1 tablespoon of ground flax seeds with 3 tablespoons of water to replace one egg in recipes. Mix the ground flax and water together in a bowl with a whisk until it becomes very gooey and gelatinous.

Chapter 6 - Which Type of Flax Should I Eat to Improve My Health?

Flaxseed oil and whole flax seed offer different benefits to health and dietary needs. Unlike ground flaxseeds, flax seed oil contains no dietary fiber at all.

Therefore, in order to really benefit from the full health benefits flax can provide, it may be better to add flaxseeds into your diet.

Whether you choose to grind the seeds down to a meal or powder, or whether you roast or toast the actual seeds to take advantage of the slightly nutty flavor, there are lots of ways you can add flax into your diet.

Whole flax seed contains 28% dietary fiber, 40% fat (with 73% of this amount made up of polyunsaturated fatty acids) and 21% protein. Other flax seed nutrients include vitamins E and B, sterols and mineral nutrients such as calcium, iron and potassium.

More than 50% of the fat in flax seed is an essential fatty acid known as Omega-3 fatty acid, (alpha-linolenic acid, or ALA). This officially makes flax seeds the richest plant source of Omega-3 fatty acid.

Add to these nutritional values the addition of being rich in antioxidants, such as lignans as other phenolic molecules and it's easy to see why flax seeds are the best option for improving your health.

Of course, there are still benefits to incorporating some flaxseed oil into your diet too, but these pale in comparison to the benefits derived by eating flax seeds.

The key is knowing how to incorporate ground flax into your diet without ruining the taste of your favorite recipes.

You can find a whole section on great tasting easy recipes later in this book.

Chapter 7 - What Are "Lignans" and Why Are They Important?

Lignans are powerful antioxidants that belong to one of the major classes of phytoestrogens. Flax is the world's best known source of lignans, which convert within our intestines into substances that are able to assist in balancing female hormones. Sesame seed is also known to contain high levels of lignans, although not in quite as concentrated amounts as flax seeds.

Research has shown that patients who have introduced flax into their diets can experience a reduction in peri-menopausal symptoms. Lignans are also thought to promote fertility.

Lignans are important for the health benefits that can be derived, particularly when it comes to cancer. Specialist research shows that when foods that are rich in lignans are eaten, they're broken down into other types of lignans by the bacteria inside the gut. From here they enter the circulation stream.

As lignans are a natural phytoestrogen with a structure that is very similar to estrogen, they have a natural affinity for the estrogen receptors found on the breasts. Yet lignans don't stimulate breast cells nearly as much as natural estrogen does. This reduces the risk of developing breast cancer by up to 58%.

Another study also showed that, in postmenopausal women who have been diagnosed with breast cancer, the mortality rate was reduced by 70% when a diet high in lignans was instigated.

The same study in postmenopausal women also showed that lignans provide a protective effect against cardiovascular disease.

With so many good reasons to include lignans into your daily diet and with flax seeds being the world's highest-known source of lignans, it's easy to see why they've become so popular.

Flax Secret 3

The Modern Disease Epidemic That Can Be Healed With Flax

The modern disease epidemic known as Type 2 diabetes was once a rare condition that affected mostly the elderly. These days it's become quite common, especially as the incidence of obesity rises within the population.

Research has shown that many diabetics also suffer from high cholesterol levels and high blood pressure. As flaxseed contains high levels of antioxidants that are helpful in reducing cholesterol levels as well as helping to control high blood pressure, this can be seen as a positive way to reduce the number of symptoms displayed by diabetics.

Flaxseeds are also beneficial in helping to regulate blood sugar levels due to the high levels of dietary fiber and massive amounts of healthy vitamins and minerals. When used in conjunction with a calorie-controlled diet, flaxseeds can be beneficial in weight loss efforts. Many studies have effectively concluded that reducing weight, especially around the abdominal region, can help to reduce dependency on insulin in diabetics.

Chapter 8 - Is Golden Flax Better Than Brown Flax?

Flax seeds are available in two basic varieties: brown and golden. Both types have very similar nutritional characteristics and both types also contain equal amounts of omega-3 fatty acids.

However, even though brown flax can be eaten in exactly the same way as golden flax and has been for thousands of years, brown flax is more commonly used as an ingredient in paint, varnish, fiber and cattle feed.

There is an exception, which is a specific variety of yellow flax seed named solin. This is sometimes labeled as Linola and it contains a completely different oil profile. It's also very low in omega-3 fatty acids, so it's not going to give the same benefits as brown or golden flaxseeds.

Regardless of whether you eat brown flax or golden flax, it is still important to drink plenty of liquids. The high dietary fiber levels in flax seeds are extremely beneficial for your health, but they could cause constipation or bowel blockages if you don't have enough fluid in your system. Drink water before your meal and you won't have this problem.

Flax Secret 4

The Right Way and the Wrong Way to Include Flax Into Your Diet

---

While it's very possible to eat raw flax seeds, or roast or toast the flaxseeds, you may be reducing some of the health benefits. This is because they are less easily digested in this form. You may find they pass right through you only partially digested.

However, if you place your flax seeds in a coffee grinder or food processor and grind them into a meal, they are far more easily digestible. Ground flax can be added to many baking recipes and can even be used as an oil alternative or even an egg alternative. There are plenty of flax recipes available to help you find more ways to add flax into your diet easily.

It's very important to store ground flax in the fridge or in the freezer, as it is perishable and may go rancid. If you prepare flax seeds improperly they will offer virtually no nutritional advantage to your body or your health. Fortunately it's very easy to prepare them correctly.

You can also use flaxseed oil in salad dressings or sauces, but it's wise not to use it as a replacement for your normal cooking oil.

Chapter 9 - Is It Safe to Eat Flax Oil?

Yes, it is very safe to eat flax oil, but it may not be safe to cook with it. Cooking with flaxseed oil isn't recommended, especially if you're thinking of just substituting your normal canola oil or vegetable oil. Trying to fry your normal recipes using flaxseed oil simply won't work.

This is because flaxseed oil breaks down at temperatures above 120F (48C). Flax oil contains high amounts of beneficial polyunsaturated fats, which are excellent for your body when they're left intact.

However when you heat flaxseed oil beyond 120F (48C), these healthy fats are destroyed, releasing free radicals instead of healthy polyunsaturated fats.

Flaxseed oil should be used cold in salad dressings for the best results.

It's important to store flaxseed in a dark place away from sunlight, as it can be affected by light. You should also remember not to keep flaxseed oil too long or it can go rancid.

If you're already adding flax seeds into your diet as a meal or just the seeds, you may not need to add extra flaxseed oil into your diet at all. This is because the seeds themselves contain the oil, so you're already receiving the benefits the oil can offer you from the seeds themselves.

If you wish to add flaxseed oil into your diet, there are some recipes for salad dressings make from flaxseed oil later in this book. You can use these to make the most of its distinctive flavor and properties.

Chapter 10 – Flax Seed Recipes

One of the biggest problems many people find after finding out how good flax can be for you is trying to figure out how to get more of it into your diet. When you start to look at some of the great recipes you can create using flax, it's much easier to find ways to include flax into your meals.

Below are some recipe suggestions that incorporate the taste and flavor of flax to full advantage.

Chicken Pot Pie

Ingredients

1 lb (500g) chicken breast, skin removed

4 cups chicken stock

1 onion

2 stalks celery

2 carrots

½ cup peas

¼ cup ground flaxseed

¼ cup plain flour

½ cup cold water

1 sheet frozen pastry (or pie crust)

Method

Cut the chicken into cubes and dice the onion, carrot and celery. Place chicken and vegetables into a large saucepan and pour chicken stock over them. Simmer over a low/medium heat for approximately an hour.

You might notice some chicken fat rising to the surface of the stock. Skim this off. Once chicken and vegetables are tender, remove them from the stock and leave to one side.

Preheat your oven to 350F (approx 180C).

In a small bowl, mix together the flour and cold water with a fork until it forms a bit of a slurry. Pour this into the broth, stirring. Return pan to the heat and continue to stir constantly until the broth mixture begins to thicken. Add chicken, vegetables, peas and flax into the broth mixture.

Spray some baking dishes with non-stick cooking spray. Spoon some of the chicken mixture into individual baking dishes.

Cut the pie crust or pastry sheet into 4 pieces and roll them into the right shape. Cover the baking dishes with pie crust.

Place baking dishes into the oven and bake them at 350F (approx 180C) for 30 minutes, or until pastry turns a lovely golden brown.

Chicken Noodle Soup

Ingredients

6 cups chicken stock

1 cup chicken meat, cut into small cubes

1 tablespoon oil

2 celery sticks, diced

1 clove garlic, crushed

½ onion, diced

1 carrot, diced

¼ cup toasted flaxseed

½ cup peas

½ cup green beans, cut into small pieces

1 cup angel-hair pasta (or vermicelli pasta)

½ teaspoon dried basil leaves

Method

In a large pot, heat oil over a medium/high heat. Add onions and garlic and sauté lightly until onion begins to soften. Add chicken stock, chicken and vegetables. Allow soup to boil for 10 minutes to soften vegetables.

Break the pasta into pieces and add to the soup. Cook for 10 minutes, until the pasta is cooked.

In a small fry pan, add ¼ cup whole flaxseed and cover with a lid. Hold the pan over a high heat, shaking it continuously so the seeds don't burn. The flaxseed should begin to pop. Continue to shake the pan over the heat until the popping stops. Your flaxseed is now toasted.

Serve the chicken noodle soup while still piping hot and garnish with a sprinkling of toasted flax seeds on each bowl.

Grandma's Flax Meatloaf

Ingredients

2 lbs (1kg) lean ground beef

1 cup skim milk

½ cup ground flax seed

½ cup dry bread crumbs

½ cup chopped onion

1 egg, lightly beaten

1 tablespoon Worcestershire sauce

1 teaspoon black pepper

1 teaspoon garlic powder

1 teaspoon dry mustard

½ teaspoon celery salt

¼ teaspoon ground thyme

½ cup ketchup

Method

Preheat your oven to 350F (180C).

In a large bowl, combine ground beef, milk, ground flax, bread crumbs, onion, egg, Worcestershire sauce, pepper, garlic powder, dry mustard, celery sale and thyme. Mix together well to ensure all ingredients are distributed through the beef.

Transfer beef mixture into a loaf pan. Lightly drizzle ketchup over the top of the loaf. Place loaf pan into the oven and bake at 350F (180C) for approximately 1 ½ hours.

Remove the pan from the oven when it's cooked and allow it to stand for 5 minutes before removing the meatloaf from the pan. Place the meatloaf onto a platter to serve immediately.

Flax Fried Rice

Ingredients

1 cup long grain rice

2 cups water

½ teaspoon salt

3 tablespoons canola oil

3 eggs, beaten

½ cup frozen peas

½ cup diced cooked ham, bacon or chicken

2 green onions

2 tablespoons soy sauce

½ teaspoon sesame oil

¼ cup toasted flaxseed

Method

Rinse rice well in a sieve under cold running water. Bring water and salt to a boil in a medium saucepan. Once water is boiling, add rice and bring back to the boil, stirring occasionally with a fork. Reduce the heat and allow rice to simmer gently for approximately 15 minutes. Much of the liquid should be absorbed by the rice by this time.

Remove from heat and place rice into a sieve. Run cold water through the rice for a few seconds to allow it to cool. This will stop the cooking process and stop your rice from going all mushy.

In a fry pan or wok, heat 1 tablespoon of canola oil over a medium heat. Add half of the beaten egg mixture and swirl it around the pan so it coats thinly. When it's almost cooked, remove it from the pan.

Roll the thin egg crepe into a tube and leave it to cool. Repeat with another tablespoon of oil and remaining egg and remove when cooked. Cut into thin strips and leave to one side for now.

Place flax seeds into a small flat pan and cover with a lid. Hold the pan over a high heat until the seeds begin to pop, remembering to shake the pan constantly to stop the seeds from burning. When the popping stops, remove from the heat and keep toasted flax seeds to one side for now.

Add another tablespoon of oil to the pan or wok and add green onions and ham or bacon. Cook until onions begin to turn soft. Add sesame oil and stir so it coats some of the ham and onion. Add rice to the pan and the peas. Cook for around 3-4 minutes, stirring ingredients through the rice. Add the soy sauce and flax seed and stir well so the rice is coated lightly by the soy sauce. Add the egg strips back into the rice. Cook for a further 3 minutes and serve immediately.

Flax Meal Tortillas

Ingredients

3 cups whole wheat flour

3 tablespoons flax meal or ground flax seeds

¼ teaspoon baking powder

1 teaspoon salt

1 tablespoon garlic powder

½ tablespoon chilli powder

3 tablespoons canola oil

1 cup warm water

Method

In a mixing bowl, mix flour, flax meal, baking powder, salt, garlic powder and chilli powder until ingredients are combined. Add canola oil and warm water and knead until the mixture forms a dough ball. If the mixture is too dry, add a little more water until a dough consistency forms.

Wrap the dough ball in saran wrap and let it stand for ten minutes.

Separate the dough into eight pieces and roll into balls. Cover each ball in saran wrap and let them stand for another ten minutes.

Roll out each ball into a ten inch round. Stack each round on plate and cover with a tea towel so they don't dry out.

Using a large griddle, preheat on range element to medium high / high. Do not grease.

Place dough round on griddle and flip it over when air pockets inside the round start to inflate. Be sure to pop the air bubbles to release the air. Tortillas are cooked when they are slightly golden in colour on both sides.

Use your tortillas immediately, or store them in refrigerator in an airtight Ziplock bag for up to five days or freeze for future use.

To use your tortillas out of the fridge or after they're defrosted: Heat, one by one, in griddle until pliable, or place one on plate, put filling in middle, and place in microwave, on high, for 15 to 20 seconds.

Gluten-Free Honey Flax Bread Rolls

Ingredients

1 ¼ cups of warm water

1 tablespoon yeast

1 teaspoon honey

2 ½ cups Almond Blend flour

¾ cup ground flaxseed

1 ½ teaspoon xanthin gum

1 teaspoon sea salt

¼ cup butter

3 tablespoons honey

2 eggs

1 teaspoon cider vinegar

Method

Mix together warm water, yeast and sugar in a small bowl. Leave to one side until mixture becomes foamy.

In a large mixing bowl, combine flour, flax, xanthin gum and salt. Using a hand mixer on a low speed, pour yeast mixture into the flour. Add butter, honey, eggs and vinegar and continue to beat on low until ingredients are combined.Once everything is well combined, increase speed on mixer to high and beat for 2 minutes.

Spray six 4-inch (10cm) cake pans with non-stick cooking spray. Measure out a heaped cup of bread mixture into each pan. Smooth out the tops with a rubber spatula. Cover pans with a kitchen towel to allow the dough to rise for 2 hours.

Preheat your oven for 375F (190C). When bread dough has risen, bake the bread rolls at 375F (190C) for 25 minutes. Remove from the oven and allow to stand for 2 minutes before turning rolls out of the pans. Leave them to cool on a wire rack before using.

Blueberry Flax Pancake

Ingredients

1 small (or ½ large) apple – roughly chopped

1 large egg

3 tablespoon flax seed meal

1 tablespoon water

1 pinch kosher or sea salt

½ cup blueberries

Method

Put the apple in a food processor or blender and pulse a few times to chop it up. Add the egg, flax seed meal, water and salt and process until well blended.

Heat a small non-stick skillet over medium high heat and spray lightly with non-stick cooking spray. Pour the batter into the hot pan and turn the heat down to low. Sprinkle the blueberries on top of the batter and gently press them into the top of the pancake.

Cook for about 6 minutes or until the edges look dry, the bottom is browned and the pancake will slide around in the pan after it has been loosened with a spatula. Flip the pancake over and cook for another 4 – 5 minutes. The pancake should feel firm to the touch. Flip onto a plate (blueberry side up) and serve. This recipe is enough to make one pancake, so it's ideal for a single-serve meal for breakfast or lunch.

Chicken Waldorf Salad with Flaxseed Oil Dressing

Ingredients

3 cups shredded cooked chicken

½ cup walnuts

2 tablespoons olive oil

2 tablespoons flaxseed oil

3 tablespoons cider vinegar

1 teaspoon honey

2 Granny Smith apples

½ cup dried cranberries

2 sticks celery

½ small red onion

Salt and pepper to taste

Method

Preheat your oven to 350F (180C). Place the walnuts onto a baking tray and toast them for about 10 minutes, or until they're crisp. Remove them from the oven and allow them to cool. When they've cooled enough, chop them roughly.

Peel the apples, remove the core and cut them into ¼ inch wedges. Chop the celery and onion finely.

In a large bowl, pour the olive oil, flaxseed oil, vinegar, honey and 2 tablespoons water. Whisk these ingredients together well. Add the apples, dried cranberries, celery, onion and chicken. Toss well to make sure the dressing is mixed over the ingredients well. Top your salad with walnuts and serve.

Banana Nut Bread

Ingredients

¾ cup ground flaxseed

2/3 cup mashed banana

½ cup white sugar

¼ cup vegetable oil

2 eggs

1 ½ cups of flour

¼ cup whole flax seeds

½ teaspoon baking powder

½ teaspoon baking soda

½ teaspoon salt

½ cup chopped walnuts

½ cup pitted dates, chopped roughly

Method

In a bowl, mix together the banana, sugar, oil and eggs at a medium speed until they're well blended.

In a separate bowl, combine the flour, ground flaxseed, whole flax seeds, baking powder, baking soda and salt. Gradually add the flour mixture into the sugar mixture and beat until they're well combined. Stir the chopped dates through the mixture.

Preheat your oven to 350F (180C).

Spray a loaf pan with non-stick cooking spray and spoon the batter into the pan. Bake the loaf at 350F (180C) for around 55-60 minutes. Test to see if loaf is fully cooked by sticking a wooden skewer into the center of the loaf. If it comes out clean, the loaf is ready.

Remove from the oven and allow to stand in the pan for 10 minutes to cool. Then turn out the loaf and allow it to cool further on a wire rack.

Spinach Bacon and Parmesan Quiche with Flax Pastry Crust

Ingredients – Pastry Crust

2 ¾ cups white flour

¼ cup ground flaxseed

1 teaspoon sea salt

2 teaspoon sugar

1 ¼ cups chilled vegetable shortening

6 tablespoons chilled water

Ingredients – Quiche Filling

2 teaspoons olive oil

1 onion, finely chopped

3.5oz (100g) chopped bacon pieces

3.5oz (100g) baby spinach leaves

4 eggs

¾ cup cream

½ cup milk

1/3 cup shredded parmesan cheese

Method – Pastry Crust

In a bowl, mix together the flour, ground flaxseed, salt and sugar. Break up the chilled vegetable shortening and cut it into the flour mixture using a fork or pastry blender until a dough is formed.

Slowly add small amounts of cold water as required in order to form a workable dough, but be careful not to overwork it. Place dough on a floured bench or board and roll the dough out. Place the dough into a lightly greased pie pan.

Preheat your oven to 425F (210C) and bake the crust for 10 minutes. Remove from the oven and leave to one side while you prepare the filling.

Method – Filling

Heat the oil in a frying pan over a medium heat. Add the onion and bacon and cook for around 8-10 minutes, or until the onion begins to soften. Remove from the heat and drain onion and bacon on a paper towel. Microwave the spinach on high for 1 minute or until it wilts. Allow to cool before squeezing out any excess moisture. Chop cooked spinach roughly.

In a mixing bowl, whisk together the eggs, cream and milk. Leave to one side for a moment.

Preheat your oven to 375F (190C).

Using your pre-prepared pastry crust, place the onion, bacon and spinach evenly over the crust. Pour the egg mixture over the fillings. Sprinkle parmesan cheese over the top and bake your quiche for 30 minutes.

Flax Chocolate Chip Cookies

Ingredients

½ cup butter

¾ cup brown sugar

¼ cup granulated sugar

2 eggs

1 ½ teaspoons vanilla essence

1 ¼ cup flour

½ cup ground flaxseed

1 teaspoon baking powder

½ teaspoon baking soda

1 teaspoon salt

2 cups chocolate chips

Method

Preheat your oven to 325F (160C)

In a bowl, cream together butter, brown sugar and granulated sugar. When the mixture is well creamed together, add two eggs and vanilla. Mix well.

In a separate bowl, mix flour, ground flaxseed, baking powder, baking soda and salt. Add the butter mixture into the flour and blend everything together well until it begins to form a dough. Stir through the chocolate chips.

Use a tablespoon to scoop the batter out into cookie-sized amounts. Place batter onto a cookie sheet around 2 inches apart, to allow them plenty of room to expand.

Bake your cookies at 325F (160C) for 12 to 15 minutes or until the cookies turn golden brown. Remove from the oven and allow the cookies to cool on the pan for a few minutes before moving them to a plate to finish cooling. Store in an airtight container until needed.

Blueberry Flax Pie

Ingredients

¾ cup white sugar

3 tablespoons cornstarch

¼ teaspoon salt

½ teaspoon ground cinnamon

1 teaspoon ground flax seed

4 cups fresh blueberries

2 pastry sheets for a 9 inch double crust pie

1 tablespoon butter

Method

Preheat your oven to 425F (220C).

In a mixing bowl, mix together the sugar, cornstarch, salt and cinnamon. Add blueberries and toss lightly to coat the blueberries in the sugar mixture.

Line a pie dish with one pie crust or pastry sheet. Pour blueberry mixture into the crust and dot with little pieces of the butter.

Cut the remaining pastry sheet into ½ inch wide strips and layer these over the blueberries to create a cross-hatch pattern.

Bake the pie on a lower shelf in your oven for approximately 50 minutes at 425F (220C), or until crust turns golden color.

Serve immediately with a scoop of vanilla ice-cream.

Apple Flax Crumble

Ingredients

3 large cooking apples, peeled and thinly sliced

1 tablespoon lemon juice

2 tablespoons white sugar

2 teaspoons white sugar

1 tablespoon cornstarch

1 ½ teaspoons ground cinnamon

1/3 cup ground flaxseed

¼ cup brown sugar

1/3 cup quick cooking oats

Method

Preheat your oven to 350F (180C).

Place sliced apples into a baking dish and pour lemon juice over them. Toss the apples lightly to coat them in the lemon.

In a small bowl, mix the sugar, cornstarch and 1 teaspoon cinnamon. Blend them well with a whisk, then pour the mixture over the apples. Toss the apples lightly once again to coat them in the mixture.

In a separate bowl, mix the flax, cinnamon, brown sugar and oats together well. Sprinkle this mixture over the apples.

Put the baking dish into the preheated oven for 40 minutes at 350F (180C). The apples should become very tender and the topping will become a lovely golden brown.

Serve immediately with a little cream, or ice cream.

Low-Fat Flax Muffins

Ingredients

½ cup whole wheat flour

1 cup plain flour (all-purpose)

¾ cup ground flaxseed

¾ cup oat bran

½ cup brown sugar

2 teaspoons baking soda

1 teaspoon baking powder

¼ teaspoon salt

2 teaspoons ground cinnamon

1 ½ cup grated carrot

½ cup raisins

2 eggs, lightly beaten

2 tablespoons applesauce

1 teaspoon vanilla essence

1 cup skim milk

1 tablespoon lemon juice

Method

Preheat your oven to 350F (180C). In a large mixing bowl, combine the flours, flax, oat bran, brown sugar, baking soda, baking powder, salt and cinnamon. Stir in grated carrot and raisins.

In a separate bowl, combine eggs, milk, lemon juice, applesauce and vanilla essence. Pour the egg mixture into the flour mixture and stir together until the dry ingredients become moist. Don't panic if the mixture looks lumpy. It will cook better this way.

Spray a muffin tin with non-stick cooking spray and pour batter into the tins. Bake the muffins for 15 to 20 minutes, or until they turn a lovely golden brown.

Green Onion Flax Salad Dressing

Ingredients

3 green onions

½ cup olive oil

½ cup flaxseed oil

1/3 cup raw apple cider vinegar

1/3 cup honey

1 ½ teaspoons sea salt

Method

Place all the ingredients into a blender and blend well until the dressing becomes creamy. Drizzle the dressing over your favorite salad ingredients.

Flaxseed Oil Dressing with Herbs

Ingredients

3 tablespoons apple cider vinegar

1 tablespoon chopped chives

1 tablespoon chopped parsley

½ teaspoon dried basil

½ teaspoon dried oregano

½ teaspoon dried mustard

1 clove garlic, chopped

3 tablespoons flaxseed oil

Pinch of cayenne pepper

Salt and pepper to taste

Method

In a food processor, combine vinegar, chives, parsley, basil, oregano, mustard and garlic, and blend until smooth. Slowly add the oil into the mixture, continuing to blend until the mixture turns slightly creamy. Season the dressing with cayenne, salt and pepper.

Drizzle the dressing over winter greens, salad greens or steamed vegetables to really bring out the flavor in this dressing.

Honey Mustard Flax Dressing

Ingredients

¼ cup apple cider vinegar

¼ cup raw honey

¼ cup flaxseed oil

¼ cup extra virgin olive oil

1 tablespoon Dijon mustard

1 clove garlic, minced

2 teaspoon dry mustard

½ teaspoon sea salt

1/8 teaspoon black pepper

Method

Place all the ingredients into a blender and blend well until the dressing becomes creamy. Serve drizzled over your favorite salad ingredients or as a sauce over steamed vegetables.

Cleansing Flax Breakfast Mix

Ingredients

1 tablespoon flax seeds

1 tablespoon sesame seeds

1 tablespoon sunflower seeds

8 almonds

1 tablespoon pumpkin seeds

1 tablespoon honey

½ cup raisins

4 tablespoons hot water

Method

Place flax seeds, sesame seeds, sunflower seeds, almonds and pumpkin seeds into a coffee grinder. Grind until they're well-mixed, or until they reach a consistency you're happy with.

Transfer ingredients into a bowl and then grind the raisins until they're soft. Add these to the bowl. Slowly add hot water, stirring. The mixture will thicken in a minute or two, so it's okay for it to be initially a little runny. Eat this mixture to help cleanse your system and boost your energy levels for the whole day.

Flax Crispy Crackers

Ingredients

2 1/2 cups whole-wheat flour

½ cup quinoa flour

2/3 cup ground golden flaxseed

1/3 cup whole flaxseed

Seasoning mix to taste (Schwartz Steakhouse pepper mix or Cajun Pepper mix)

1 ½ cups warm water

Method

Put the whole-wheat flour, ground flaxseed, whole flaxseed and the seasoning mix of your choice into a food mixer. Blend ingredients together for about 15 seconds

Add all the warm water and mix well for about 1 minute.

Make sure the dough is not too sticky or too dry. Add water or flour to adjust the consistency. Put the mixture aside to rest for ½ hour. Roll out the mixture and using a cookie cutter cut out the crackers.

Place on a greased cooking tin or baking sheet and bake for 8 to ten minutes at 350F (180C) or until golden brown.

Store cookies in an air tight biscuit tin. Use with dips and sauces as a snack.

Savoury Flax Pancakes

Ingredients

1 cup sweet potato

1 cup carrots

2 tabelspoon fresh parsley

1 large egg

¼ cup whole-wheat flour

¼ cup round Flaxseed

1 teaspoon baking powder

1 small chili pepper

¼ cup milk

2 tablespoons melted butter

Virgin Olive Oil for cooking

Method

In a mixing bowl, grate the sweet potato and carrots, and chop the fresh parsley finely. Combine with the egg and mix well. Add all the remaining ingredients and combine thoroughly.

Pour a small amount of olive oil into a frying pan and heat it over a medium heat. Reduce the heat to medium/low. Drop 1 tablespoon of the batter mix into the frying pan. Cook for 2-3 minutes over a gentle heat. Turn over the pancake and cook the other side for a further minute or so.

Serve with pickle, cottage cheese or lumpy mango chutney

Chapter 11 – Raw Flax V Cooked Flax

There are a variety of ways to add flax into your diet. Flax oil is easily available and ground flax can be added to other foods. But what's the right way to add these things into your diet?

While there are plenty of specific flax recipes available, sometimes it's very possible to substitute another ingredient for ground flax or toasted flax seeds. In other cases, it's very possible to add ground flax into other foods.

For example, you can easily add a tablespoon or so of ground flax into your morning juice or even into a glass of chocolate milk.

You're able to sprinkle ground flax onto your cereal in the morning, or you can add ground flax into yogurt.

Flax as an Oil Substitute

When used as a substitute ingredient, you can adapt any of your current favorite recipes to include more flax. If your recipe requires 1/3 cup of oil, replace this with 1 cup of ground flaxseed instead. This is a 3:1 substitution.

Flax as an Egg Substitute

There are other recipes that call for eggs to bind specific ingredients together. If this is the case, simply mix 1 tablespoon of ground flax seeds with 3 tablespoons of water to replace one egg in recipes. Mix the ground flax and water together in a bowl with a whisk until it becomes very gooey and gelatinous. If you need two eggs in a particular recipe, simply double the portions of ground flax seeds and water.

This will have a similar texture to egg whites and will work very well in many recipes, especially for vegans who may want to replace eggs in their favorite recipes.

Keep in mind that if a recipe requires both eggs and vegetable oil, it's wise to substitute only one or the other of these options. Trying to substitute both could give you an incorrect consistency and an incorrect cooking time with variable results.

Flax as a Flour Substitute

For recipes that require flour, reduce the amount of flour you need by 25% and replace it with the same portion of ground flaxseed. So if your recipe requires 1 cup of flour, change this so you're putting in ¾ cup of flour and ¼ cup of ground flaxseed instead. You should find that you won't even taste the flax seed in most recipes, while some recipes are specifically created to enhance and highlight the nutty taste of the flax.

Differences in Flax for Baking

Always remember that if you're using ground flax in your baking, you may find your recipes may turn brown more quickly, so it's important to monitor your baking so it won't burn. You may also find that you might need to adjust the baking temperature a little from the original recipe.

The best way to determine what works in your own baking recipes is to keep a careful eye on your oven while your goods are cooking. When your goods are ready, take a note of the time it took to complete and make a note of this next to your original recipe. You should also make a note of how much flax you used to substitute your chosen ingredients.

This way you'll have notes to remind you of the changes you made. You'll also be able to repeat the recipe again at the right temperature and right cooking time without having to guess.

Flax Secret 5

How to Prepare and Eat Flax Raw

It's possible to simply sprinkle whole flax seed onto salads, oatmeal, rice, yogurt, beans sandwiches and cereals. In fact, you can create your own breakfast cereal from flax, as long as you get the right blend of ingredients. This can be an excellent cleansing cereal that will help boost your energy and flush toxins from your system.

You can also add whole flax seed to creamed potatoes. Simply stir them into the potatoes to blend them well. The slightly nutty flavor can enhance the flavor of the potatoes. Flax seed can also be added to milkshakes and smoothies. If you prefer to add flax into other foods and recipes, put some seeds into a coffee grinder or food blender and grind them into a meal. Use the ground flax seed as a replacement for cooking oil. 1 ½ cups of ground flax seed is equivalent to ½ cup of cooking oil.

You can also use ground flax as an egg replacement in your regular recipes by adding 1 tablespoon of ground flax and 3 tablespoons of water to create a gelatinous mixture to use in place of eggs.

Conclusion

There is such a diverse range of health benefits to including a little flax into your diet. There are also enormous numbers of great recipes you can try in order to introduce more flax seed into your diet.

While some of the recipes are very quick and simple, some may require a little practice and patience to get them right. The key is to work on ways to continue eating the foods you enjoy the most while still incorporating a little flax seed into those original recipes without changing the taste too much.

You can choose to toast your flax seeds and sprinkle them over other recipes to take advantage of the nutty taste. You might prefer to grind your flax seeds into a meal and use them in the actual recipes. You can even include a little flaxseed oil in your salad dressing to help increase the amount of ALA you get into your diet.

No matter what option you choose, you should notice the health benefits within a very short time.

Here's to better health and a happier life.

Resources

You can find the latest information on flax on the accompanying website to this book. There are free recipes that I will be developing. There are reports and videos keeping you up to date on the latest research and information on eating seeds and grains.

www.flaxtips.com

My other site is all about the superfood quinoa

www.quinoatips.com

I have a weekly newsletter that is sent by email. You can sign up at the following website

www.takehealthaction.com

About The Author

Ken Jones is an author and writer on how to include seeds and grains into your daily diet. His Quinoa Cookbook was published in December 2009. It has become one of the top selling books in the food sections of the major online retailers.

This companion volume follows in the same way by providing information on why you should eat Flax and making the eating of Flax a simple process.

Other Title By The Same Author

The Quinoa Cookbook – ISBN 978-1449583583.